The Sculptor

The gnarled, beaten lump of wood,

disregarded and ignored for many years,

finally gets noticed, picked up and studied.

A twinkling in the sculptors eyes,

raises the hope for the wood.

It has purpose, usefulness,

not to be just thrown on the fire,

to burn into ashes and then forgotten.

Expert fingers run up and down the bark,

gently feeling the knots and chips.

So the sculptor begins, slowly at first,

so as not to ruin the idea forming in his head.

Flaking away loose bits and peeling the bark.

It is not a quick task, to hasten could ruin the outcome.

Then the chisel is used, again gently and precisely

a shape slowly forming.

Sometimes the wood feels pain, but it knows it isn't permanent,

and suffers, knowing that the outcome will make it all worthwhile.

Many weeks pass, the wood slowly taking shape.

The sculptor often pausing, to reassess his plan,

feeling the wood as its rough skin starts to smoothen.

The shape is in his mind, forming, evolving.

The wood is becoming more aware of its new shape,

It's new beginning.

It is pleased with the new shape forming,

feeling re-energised, having a purpose, a future.

Weeks turn to months, the sculptor is pleased with his progress,

But, is also aware he needs to stop.

The sculpture is not complete,

however, it is the turn of his apprentice now.

There is still much to do, but he is confident in his apprentices'
understanding and ability.

The wood, feeling hopeful, has some trepidation,

with the thought of new hands moulding it.

Will it be hurt more? Ruined by the slip of the chisel?

But, it also has confidence in the sculptors' vision.

At last it is finished, the apprentice made a few errors,

there were a few slips of the chisel.

But, overall, the work is complete,

the wood now smooth and silky.

It is pleased with its new shape, new identity.

Thank you for not tossing me into the fire,

but taking the time and attention to smooth my rough edges,

seeing something worthwhile deep inside,

After The Storm

The storm is finally abating,

it seems like it was raging for hours,

The crashing waves shattering the ship.

The water over my head, drowning, no way out,

Struggling to make sense, wanting to sink,

another body on the seabed.

But knowing the lifeboat is there,

Clambering in, exhausted after hours of exertion.

But, probably no more than just one hour,

no energy left, eyes red and swollen,

tears still falling onto the pillow,

but slower, body relaxing, brain starting to function.

Needing sleep, to rebuild the energy,

calm the thoughts, be able to focus.

Waves now just lap gently against the side of the life boat.

No oars to use, no direction thought of,

just laying, bobbing up and down,

being rocked by the sea.

The smell and tang of the salty water,

the feel of the breeze,

but no sounds, not yet,

those will come later,

for now there is no noise, just peace,

being rocked gently off to sleep.

Once awake, there will be more focus,

noises slowly allowed to enter the ears,

the body, will not be so stiff and achy,

and be able to move without thought.

But, for now there are no oars,

no land in the distance

just peace and calm,

peace and calm.

Body relaxing, eyes drying,

twisted mess, unravelling , thoughts not racing,

but, recognisable, understandable, not attacking,

just suggesting, sparking, idling.

The shipwreck just a memory.

Then land is sighted,

A course plotted,

Oars appear, and sounds are noticed.

The overwhelming wave of despair,

calmed, over for now.

The functioning brain slowly making sense,

Slowly evolving a plan, simple, easy.

Nothing to cause another storm.

Not yet.

The realisation of how many storms have gone past

That more will come,

Maybe rougher, maybe not.

But maybe there will be an inkling of hope

That the lifeboat, then land will appear again.

If Only

Bobbing up and down with the waves,

sun glistening on the salty water.

Calm and peaceful.

Seagulls above, sand and fish below,

waves splashing onto the rocks or escaping up the drying sand.

Calm and peaceful.

Kids splashing and playing,

laughing and screaming, but still,

calm and peaceful.

If only I could press pause, and languish in the calm,

for just a few moments more.

If only

all my other thoughts would behave , queue up in an orderly fashion,

wait their turn, no pushing or shoving.

If only

my thoughts weren't an angry mob,

chasing and shouting at me, trapping me against a wall.

If only

life would challenge me with one thing at a time,

manageable and not demanding.

If only

my head wasn't a messy ball of wool,

with ends sticking out everywhere, a tangled mess.

My head, my life.

Calm and peaceful.

If only.......

Death

An empty chasm, bottomless, never-ending,

Dark and forbidding, it engulfs.

A pillow pressed hard over mouth and nose,

struggling for breath, the fight continues.

Dizziness, feeling feint, not knowing when the struggle will end,

So slowly the time passes.

Muffled sounds of others, trying to help,

Trying to understand, to take the pain away.

The pain seems endless, the voices distant and meaningless.

Like an amputation, there seems no remedy.

The death of anyone human or animal.

Crushes the chest, restricting the lungs.

Breaking the heart, making life so difficult.

Not just a death, a heart wrenching, wailing,

Inconsolable death.

Never to see, feel, hear, hug again.

Just a big void.

Memories remain, happy times.

But, the sadness also continues,

acceptance starts to gain momentum.

The hurt lessens, the emotions stabilise.

Breathing becomes easier.

The pressure on the pillow lessens,

energy to fight the suffocation increases.

The muffled voices become clearer.

The words now have meaning.

Can be understood, appreciated.

The chasm is still there,

But now there is a bridge starting to form.

A ladder reaching to the top,

A way up, out, across.

With acceptance and time, the chasm is surmountable.

Isn't such a challenge, can be faced and conquered.

The pillow, shrinks, allowing breathing once again.

Time returns to normal.

Allowing slots for remembrance and sorrow,

But also for happiness, joy and hope.

Life resumes, but memories remain

R.I.P. xx

Bad Winter

Fairy lights twinkling like electric shocks.

Carols in every shop, sound like nails scraping down a blackboard.

Wrapped presents are an avalanche engulfing and suffocating me.

People everywhere with bags full of presents,

Claustrophobia washes over me like a tidal wave.

Relief when Christmas is finished,

The paper rotting in the recycling,

The lights and decorations, back in their boxes,

shoved as far back on the shelf as possible.

No more putting on a happy face

Having to hide the thoughts and memories haunting me

Then the new year,

just another day.

The day after yesterday.

Resolutions which will be broken in a matter of weeks.

More thoughts and memories follow.

Chasing after me like a pack of wolves,

No hiding from them.

They will catch me in the end.

They always do.

Ripping and tearing, sharp claws and fangs.

The memories drawing blood once again.

There's no escape, the wolves do not tire.

But I do, the resistance lessens.

Tunnel visioned I seek my normal exit.

Knowing deep down that I need help,

But still I buy, hoard, then swallow.

I need to tell, but want to die.

I have no understanding of why it matters.

No comprehension why people worry.

I am no use to anyone, I am a burden.

An inconvenience to eradicate.

Apathy overcomes me,

no energy to fight.

I admit my actions.

Get treatment,

Knowing resistance is futile.

A weight is lifted from my shoulders.

But I am still haunted.

Still the wolves rip at me.

Wanting now to know answers.

Why all the fuss?

Why does it matter so much?

I don't deserve this attention.

I am confused, bewildered.

Why does everyone insist I should live

When I want the opposite.

Why do I have to keep being punished.

The questions tear at my flesh in a frenzy.

But no answers that make sense are forthcoming.

So the pain and torture remains, unsolved.

Broken Heart

The stomach churning feeling of uselessness.

Rears its ugly head,

Taunting my every thought,

My every word and action.

What is there to say?

How to console, to take the pain away?

Long ago a kiss would make the hurt better,

But how to kiss a broken heart better?

Each time it hurts just like the first time.

If there was anyway to take the pain away,

To swap her heart with mine.

I would do it in a heartbeat.

But all I can do is hug, listen,

murmur and repeat consoling phrases.

To try and understand the pain,

just like the first time.

One phrase keeps being repeated,

'Why cant I be like you and dad?'

Childhood sweethearts.

Still together after all these years.

We both have had our share of broken hearts,

But it is always so raw,

life can never be the same.

But after the initial shock,

With good friends and family support.

It will become less painful,

Maybe next time it wont end in a broken heart.

Maybe next time it wont end.

Cat

Cutely curled up, one front paw on his tail,

the other tucked neatly under his whiskery chin.

The cat seems in a deep sleep,

But one part of him is always awake, alert.

He still hears, smells, feels for prey or attacker.

He is ready to pounce.

But for now he just looks cute,

Shiny, soft, deep fur, big paws relaxed.

All of a sudden he jumps,

Clawing at self worth, biting through concentration and hope,

shredding sleep and appetite, ripping motivation and energy into tiny bits.

But all the time nudging and shaping the swelling,

'everyone would be better off with you dead, ' it throbs.

Enjoyment oozes out of every cut, lost forever.

Red angry suicide envelops every open wound.

The silent killer rests for a while,

Purring in satisfaction at the pain and suffering it has inflicted.

But not content quite yet.

Cleaning and sharpening his claws in readiness.

The fat, fluffy, fur bag, rolls onto his back,

Legs apart, waiting for the all too tempting tummy rub.

And so the next onslaught begins.

Front paws grasping, strong, muscular hind legs causing the damage.

The prey is trapped and the cat doesn't give up,

Until there is nothing left,

apart from the swelling growing bigger,

'you need to die,' it throbs.

The cat is content for now,

If the brain he rests on, gives in to the swelling

Then, he will find another vulnerable one,

If not, his claws and teeth are still sharp,

He will not give in,

He will play for a while longer.

And then go for the kill.

All the while, the cute paws, soft fur,

Huge round eyes, eminate vulnerability and tameness.

But depression just purrs, biding his time.

It Will Pass

Deep dark pit, despair,

struggling from one minute to the next,

trying to keep going, struggling to just exist.

Minuscule tasks sap every drop of strength,

no energy, everything a challenge,

no joy, no fun, just existing

It WILL pass

Mountain peak, bright, sunny,

exhilaration, crisp fresh air.

Sun rays bouncing off the rocks and slipping into crevices.

Enjoying the moment, energy, concentration,

feeling alive, happiness, seeing and feeling.

Joy, fun, a sense of hope.

Unfortunately, it too will pass.

Deep dark pit or top of the mountain?

So difficult to be aware of one when at the other.

Like ships in the night they silently pass,

neither ever aware of the other.

One day there will be a meadow to cushion the impending fall,

from peak to pit.

One day there will be a ladder to the meadow,

from the pit.

One day there will be an easier path to the apex,

from the meadow.

After the meadow will come more landscapes,

more levels to understand,

and quench the never ending thirst to climb,

to give more energy, more life, just more.

There will be snakes that slide downwards,

But, the landscapes will help ease the fall.

Give hope that the climb wont be such a task,

the fall not so far, the mountain achievable once again.

One day there will be sand beneath your feet,

there will be birds singing in the trees.

You will hear the waves crashing against the shore,

you will smell the sweet scent of cut grass,

you will feel the crunch of fresh snow beneath your feet.

There will no longer be the tremendous effort

needed to struggle between apex and abyss.

One day there will be awareness of all landscapes,

good and bad.

There will be no ships silently passing,

just waves overlapping seamlessly,

and then you will understand that it will pass.

Waterfall

Ice melting, slowly trickling its way down the mountain,

eroding more of the rock as it picks up speed,

its haste to get to the sea, a long way off.

The trickle becomes a stream, then a river,

Getting faster and more forceful, as it rushes on.

Until,

The water crashes down in a frenzy, foaming in its haste,

Desperate, to carry on its journey,

To reach the rocks, create the whirlpools,

Tumbling in fury, trying to fly.

Then the drop, sudden, jolting, freedom,

droplets catching the sun, creating beautiful seabows.

Colours brightly shining, shadowing the droplets fall.

Many coloured arcs, dancing in the air,

to a tune only they can hear,

Rehearsed over thousands of years.

The waterfall, so stunning, beautiful, enticing.

The deafening roar,

the deadly currents seeming so innocent.

Racing on to the next flight of freedom,

The next deadly drop, spraying over the top,

Breeze and Sun, catching the droplets once again.

The jagged rocks, rising from the river bed,

Gasping for air, catching the water off guard.

Sending it swirling in all directions,

Once again tumbling and dancing down the river.

Suddenly there's peace, the raging rapids now a gentle river,

Being guided by the river banks, abundant with stones and pebbles,

Smoothed over millennium.

Meandering slowly, separating the land,

Giving sustenance to the animals dependent upon it.

Keeping the fauna alive, to give the vibrant luscious green glow.

For miles in every direction.

None of it realising the rivers previous perilous journey.

Tofly

The address written in scribbled rushed handwriting,

The stamp carelessly put in the corner,

shoved into the post box, without a second thought.

The envelope fell a short way and landed awkwardly on top of the pile.

It was dark, smelly, crowded and scarey in the box.

Soon more letters and parcels piled on top.

Just as the envelope thought he was going to suffocate,

There was a loud jangling of keys and the box opened.

Fresh air and rain blew fiercely through the opening.

The mesh basket was roughly yanked from the box,

and turned upside down,

the contents spilling into the big sack.

The sack was then chucked into the back of the smelly van.

The envelope was picked on by the bullying parcels,

Throwing their weight around,

The birthday cards ignored him,

The bills and final demands just laughed at him.

The envelope was all alone, and was feeling very sad.

He didn't know what to do, he knew he had to wait,

the envelope had a special task, and couldn't give up.

Just because he wasn't the same as any of them,

they picked on him.

It was when the recorded delivery letters started jumping on him,

Crumpling his edges and causing a couple of rips,

he knew he couldn't wait any longer.

It was payback time.

All of the letters and envelopes bullied previously,

Just because they were slightly different.

it was his mission to make the bullies realise,

To make them understand.

Sacrifice the one for the many, he had been told.

He would be a martyr,

He would be remembered for his sacrifice.

So it was time, the red, angry, suicide envelope looked around,

he was nervous but, knew he was the chosen one,

He took a deep breath and blew open the seal,

his contents showering all the nasty letters and parcels.

There was screaming and shouting from the post,

As they all were covered in the dreaded green ink.

the ink which means they go into the unknown sack,

Never to be delivered.

As the red, angry, suicide envelope lay dying,

He was happy that all the post now looked the same,

no pecking order, they all looked alike.

He had made his statement, and done it well.

All the post was now tree frog green.

Then as he lay dying, the post heard him cry out:

'Total oneness for letters, yippee',

Which became known as 'tofly',

whenever there was the slightest hint of bullying,

'Tofly' would be said.

So that all the post remembered and lived in harmony.

www.ingramcontent.com/pod-product-compliance
Lightning Source LLC
Chambersburg PA
CBHW021450170526
45164CB00001B/457